LOW GLYCEMIC INDEX FOODS LIST

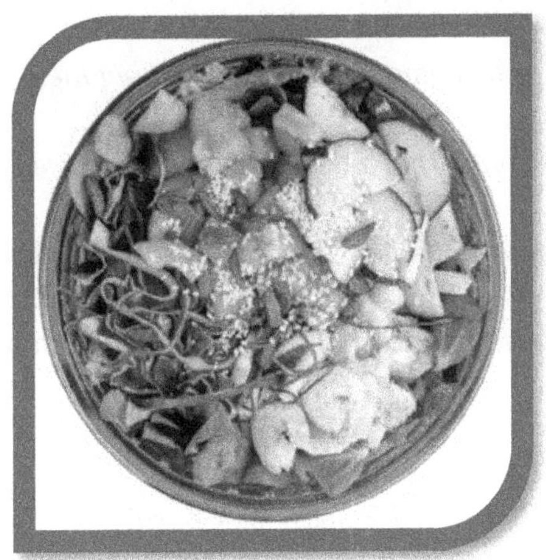

The Ultimate Guide to a GI Diet for Easy Diabetes Meal Planning and Healthy Eating.

ARIA G JAMES

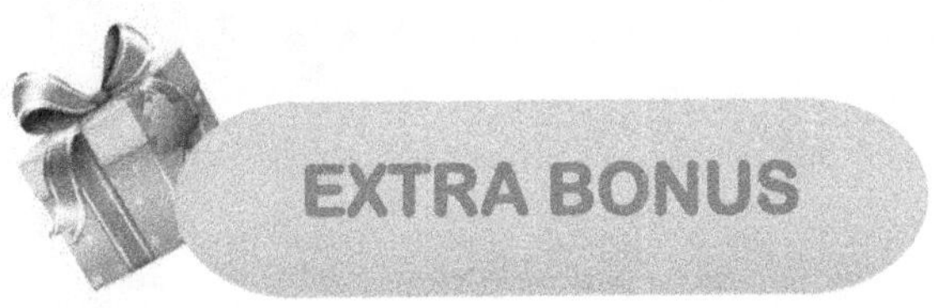

BONUS 1:

20 RECIPES FOR

HEALTHY EATING

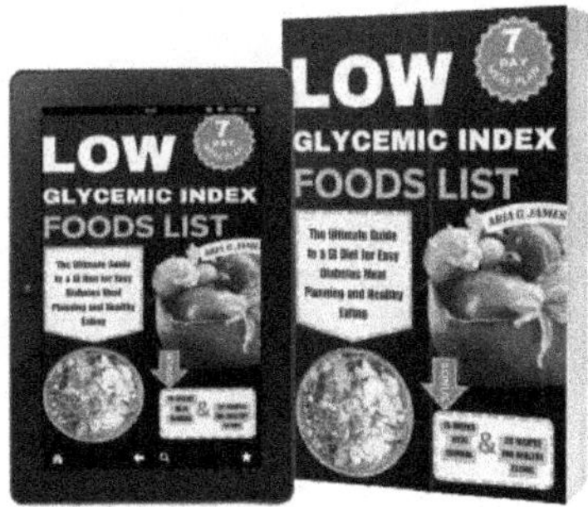

BONUS 2:

10-WEEKS

MEAL JOURNAL

SCAN THE QR CODE BELOW TO GAIN MORE BOOKS FROM THIS AUTHOR.

TABLE OF CONTENTS

INTRODUCTION

Welcome to "Low Glycemic Index Foods List: The Ultimate Guide to a GI Diet for Easy Diabetes Meal Planning and Healthy Eating"

In today's fast-paced world, where convenience often takes precedence over health, our relationship with food has a significant impact on our well-being. The prevalence of diabetes and the increasing need for dietary strategies to manage blood sugar levels have underscored the importance of understanding how the foods we eat affect our bodies.

This comprehensive guide aims to demystify the concept of the glycemic index (GI) and its implications for our dietary choices, especially for individuals managing diabetes or those seeking to adopt healthier eating habits. The glycemic index categorizes foods based on how quickly they raise blood sugar levels. By incorporating low GI foods into our diets, we can stabilize blood sugar, improve energy levels, and promote overall health.

Within the pages of this book, you'll find a wealth of knowledge distilled into easily understandable sections. We'll delve into the fundamental principles of the glycemic index, explore the benefits of a low GI diet, and provide you with an extensive list of foods categorized by their glycemic index values. Moreover, we'll equip you with practical meal plans, tantalizing recipes, and tips for integrating these wholesome foods into your daily routine effortlessly.

Whether you're seeking to manage diabetes more effectively, striving for sustained energy levels throughout the day, or simply aiming to make informed choices for your health, this book is designed to be your go-to resource. It's a tool crafted to empower you with the knowledge and inspiration needed to embrace a lifestyle centered around nutritious, low GI foods.

So, join us on this enlightening journey toward better health and vitality. Let's embark together on a path that celebrates the nourishing power of low glycemic index foods and enables you to make mindful, delicious choices that will fuel your well-being.

Here's to a healthier, happier you!

UNDERSTANDING THE GLYCEMIC INDEX

Understanding the Glycemic Index (GI) is pivotal in comprehending the relationship between food and its impact on blood sugar levels. It serves as a critical tool in managing various health conditions, especially diabetes, and optimizing overall well-being. This comprehensive guide aims to unravel the intricacies of the GI, exploring its definition, influence on blood sugar levels, and the myriad benefits of incorporating low GI foods into one's diet.

❖ **What is the Glycemic Index?**

The Glycemic Index is a ranking system that assigns a numerical value to carbohydrates based on their effect on blood glucose levels after consumption. It classifies foods on a scale of 0 to 100, with higher values indicating a more rapid increase in blood sugar levels.

❖ **The Impact of GI on Blood Sugar Levels**

When carbohydrates are consumed, they are broken down into glucose, which enters the bloodstream and affects blood sugar levels.

Foods with a high GI value cause a rapid spike in blood glucose levels, prompting the pancreas to release a surge of insulin to regulate this increase. This swift rise in blood sugar is common in foods like white bread, sugary snacks, and processed cereals.

Conversely, low GI foods are digested and absorbed more slowly, leading to a gradual increase in blood glucose levels. This slower, more controlled release of glucose results in a steadier and more sustained energy supply. Low GI foods include most fruits and vegetables, legumes, whole grains like oats and barley, and specific dairy products.

❖ **Benefits of Low GI Foods**

The incorporation of low GI foods into one's diet offers a plethora of advantages that extend beyond blood sugar control:

Blood Sugar Management: One of the most significant benefits of low GI foods is their ability to help manage blood sugar levels effectively. For individuals with diabetes or those aiming to prevent insulin spikes, consuming a diet rich in low GI foods can aid in maintaining stable blood glucose levels throughout the day.

Sustained Energy Release: Low GI foods provide a sustained and consistent release of energy. This steady supply of energy helps in avoiding energy crashes and feelings of fatigue commonly associated with consuming high GI foods. It also supports enhanced endurance during physical activities.

Weight Management: Incorporating low GI foods into one's diet can aid in weight management. These foods typically have higher fiber content and promote a feeling of fullness, reducing the likelihood of overeating and helping individuals control their calorie intake.

Improved Heart Health: Research suggests that a diet comprising predominantly low GI foods may contribute to better heart health. It can potentially lower the risk of heart disease by improving lipid profiles, reducing inflammation, and managing other risk factors associated with cardiovascular issues.

Understanding the Glycemic Index empowers individuals to make informed dietary choices that align with their health goals. By prioritizing low GI foods, individuals can foster better blood sugar control, sustained energy levels, and overall well-being.

❖ Incorporating Low GI Foods into Your Diet

Transitioning to a diet centered around low GI foods doesn't necessitate a complete overhaul. Simple modifications, such as swapping refined grains for whole grains, choosing fresh fruits and vegetables over processed snacks, and opting for lean protein sources, can significantly impact blood sugar regulation and overall health.

Moreover, meal planning that includes a balance of low GI foods, such as incorporating quinoa, sweet potatoes, leafy greens, and beans can result in diverse, flavorful, and nourishing meals.

Understanding the Glycemic Index serves as a cornerstone in making informed dietary choices. By prioritizing low GI foods, individuals can manage blood sugar levels effectively, sustain energy levels, and promote overall health and well-being. Incorporating these foods into a balanced diet not only aids in managing diabetes but also offers an array of health benefits that contribute to a healthier, more vibrant life.

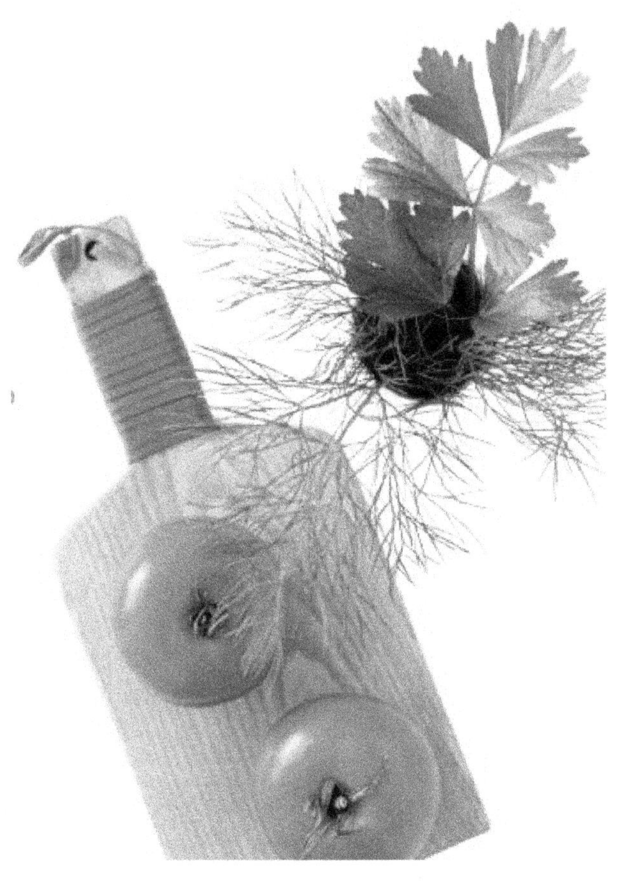

Understanding the basics of a Glycemic Index (GI) diet is fundamental to harnessing the benefits of low GI foods for improved health and well-being. This section, will delve into the principles of a low GI diet, the utilization of the Glycemic Index for meal planning, and the pivotal importance of carbohydrate quality in promoting better health outcomes.

❖ **Principles of a Low GI Diet**

A Low GI diet centers around consuming foods that rank lower on the Glycemic Index scale. The primary principles include:

Choosing Low GI Foods: Prioritizing foods with a low GI value, typically 55 or less, forms the foundation of this diet. These include most fruits and vegetables, whole grains, legumes, and certain dairy products.

Balancing Carbohydrates: Focusing on the quality and quantity of carbohydrates consumed is crucial. Instead of entirely eliminating carbs, the emphasis lies on selecting complex carbohydrates, which digest more slowly and have a lower impact on blood sugar levels.

Pairing with Proteins and Healthy Fats: Combining low GI carbohydrates with lean proteins and healthy fats can further mitigate blood sugar spikes and enhance satiety.

Portion Control and Frequency: Moderation and mindful portion control are key. Spreading out meals and snacks evenly throughout the day helps maintain stable blood sugar levels.

❖ Utilizing the Glycemic Index for Meal Planning

Integrating the Glycemic Index into meal planning involves a systematic approach:

Understanding GI Values: Familiarizing oneself with the GI values of various foods is essential. Reference tables or online resources provide comprehensive lists detailing the GI rankings of numerous foods.

Building Balanced Meals: Crafting meals with a combination of low GI foods, lean proteins, healthy fats, and a variety of colorful fruits and vegetables is key. For instance, a meal might include quinoa (low GI), grilled chicken (protein), and a side of steamed broccoli (low GI vegetable).

Creating Snack Options: Opting for low GI snacks, such as Greek yogurt with berries or whole-grain crackers with hummus, can help maintain steady blood sugar levels between meals.

Adjusting Cooking Methods: Altering cooking techniques, like opting for steaming or roasting instead of frying, can influence a food's GI. For instance, boiled sweet potatoes have a lower GI than fried sweet potato chips.

❖ **Importance of Carbohydrate Quality**

Carbohydrates play a significant role in the Glycemic Index and overall health. The quality of carbohydrates matters more than merely the quantity:

Differentiating Between Simple and Complex Carbs: Simple carbohydrates, found in refined grains and sugars, tend to have a higher GI and can cause rapid spikes in blood sugar levels. In contrast, complex carbohydrates, present in whole grains, legumes, and fibrous fruits and vegetables, have a lower GI, digest more slowly, and provide sustained energy.

Favoring Fiber-Rich Foods: Foods high in fiber, such as whole grains, nuts, seeds, fruits, and vegetables, not only have a lower GI but also aid in digestion, promote satiety, and contribute to overall gut health.

Impact on Health: High-quality carbohydrates, particularly those with a lower GI, contribute to better blood sugar control, reduced risk of chronic diseases like diabetes and heart disease, and improved overall health outcomes.

Incorporating these principles into daily life fosters a balanced approach to nutrition, supporting stable blood sugar levels, sustained energy, weight management, and overall well-being.

The basics of a Glycemic Index diet revolve around making informed food choices that prioritize low GI foods, emphasize balanced meal planning, and recognize the significance of carbohydrate quality.

FRUITS:

Cherries

GI Value: 22

GL Value: 6

Portion Size: 1 cup (about 21 cherries)

Preparation: Enjoy cherries as a snack, in salads, or as a topping for yogurt.

Grapefruit

GI Value: 25

GL Value: 3

Portion Size: ½ medium fruit

Preparation: Eat grapefruit as is or include it in fruit salads.

Apples

GI Value: 39

GL Value: 6

Portion Size: 1 medium apple

Preparation: Have apples whole or sliced with nut butter as a snack.

Pears

GI Value: 38

GL Value: 4

Portion Size: 1 medium pear

Preparation: Enjoy pears fresh or add them to salads and baked dishes.

Plums

GI Value: 24

GL Value: 3

Portion Size: 2 medium plums

Preparation: Eat plums as a snack or add them to yogurt or oatmeal.

Berries (e.g., Strawberries, Blueberries, Raspberries)

GI Value: Varies (Generally low)

GL Value: Varies

Portion Size: 1 cup (varies by type)

Preparation: Enjoy berries fresh, add them to smoothies, or top cereals with them.

Oranges

GI Value: 40

GL Value: 5

Portion Size: 1 medium orange

Preparation: Eat oranges whole or use their segments in salads.

Apricots

GI Value: 34

GL Value: 4

Portion Size: 3 whole apricots

Preparation: Enjoy fresh apricots as a snack or add them to yogurt.

Kiwi

GI Value: 47

GL Value: 7

Portion Size: 1 medium kiwi

Preparation: Eat kiwi as is or add it to fruit salads.

Peaches

GI Value: 42

GL Value: 5

Portion Size: 1 medium peach

Preparation: Enjoy fresh peaches or use them in smoothies.

VEGETABLES:

Spinach

GI Value: 15

GL Value: 0

Portion Size: 1 cup (raw)

Preparation: Use spinach in salads, sandwiches, or sauté as a side dish.

Broccoli

GI Value: 10

GL Value: 1

Portion Size: 1 cup (cooked)

Preparation: Steam or roast broccoli as a side dish or add it to stir-fries.

Cauliflower

GI Value: 15

GL Value: 2

Portion Size: 1 cup (raw)

Preparation: Enjoy cauliflower raw with dip or roast it as a side dish.

Green Beans

GI Value: 15

GL Value: 2

Portion Size: 1 cup (cooked)

Preparation: Steam or stir-fry green beans as a side dish.

Zucchini

GI Value: 15

GL Value: 2

Portion Size: 1 cup (cooked)

Preparation: Grill, sauté, or bake zucchini as a side dish or in casseroles.

Asparagus

GI Value: 15

GL Value: 1

Portion Size: 1 cup (cooked)

Preparation: Steam, roast, or grill asparagus for a nutritious side dish.

Bell Peppers

GI Value: 15

GL Value: 1

Portion Size: 1 cup (raw)

Preparation: Use raw bell peppers in salads or roast them as a side dish.

Cabbage

GI Value: 10

GL Value: 1

Portion Size: 1 cup (raw)

Preparation: Use cabbage in salads, coleslaw, or stir-fries.

Carrots

GI Value: 39

GL Value: 2

Portion Size: 1 medium carrot

Preparation: Enjoy carrots raw with dip or add them to soups and salads.

Tomatoes

GI Value: 15

GL Value: 1

Portion Size: 1 medium tomato

Preparation: Use tomatoes fresh in salads or sandwiches, or cook them in sauces.

❖ **Glycemic Grains and Cereals**

GRAINS:

Barley

GI Value: 28

GL Value: 12

Portion Size: ½ cup (cooked)

Preparation: Cook barley in water or broth, use as a side dish or in soups and salads.

Bulgur

GI Value: 48

GL Value: 12

Portion Size: ½ cup (cooked)

Preparation: Cook bulgur in boiling water, use in pilafs, salads, or as a base for stuffed vegetables.

Quinoa

GI Value: 53

GL Value: 13

Portion Size: ½ cup (cooked)

Preparation: Rinse quinoa, cook in water or broth, use as a versatile base for different dishes.

Brown Rice

GI Value: 50

GL Value: 16

Portion Size: ½ cup (cooked)

Preparation: Rinse rice, cook in water, serve as a side dish, or in stir-fries and casseroles.

Wild Rice

GI Value: 57

GL Value: 18

Portion Size: ½ cup (cooked)

Preparation: Cook wild rice in water, use in salads, pilafs, or as a side dish.

Pearl Barley

GI Value: 25

GL Value: 11

Portion Size: ½ cup (cooked)

Preparation: Cook pearl barley, use in soups, stews, or as a base for grain bowls.

Whole Grain Spelt

GI Value: 54

GL Value: 17

Portion Size: ½ cup (cooked)

Preparation: Cook spelt, use in salads, soups, or as a side dish.

Amaranth

GI Value: 46

GL Value: 11

Portion Size: ½ cup (cooked)

Preparation: Cook amaranth, use as a porridge, in soups, or as a side dish.

Millet

GI Value: 71

GL Value: 23

Portion Size: ½ cup (cooked)

Preparation: Cook millet in water or broth, use in pilafs, as a side dish, or in baked goods.

Farro

GI Value: 40

GL Value: 15

Portion Size: ½ cup (cooked)

Preparation: Cook farro, use in salads, soups, or as a side dish.

Rolled Oats

GI Value: 55

GL Value: 11

Portion Size: ½ cup (cooked)

Preparation: Cook rolled oats in water or milk, add fruits or nuts for a nutritious breakfast.

Steel-Cut Oats

GI Value: 55

GL Value: 11

Portion Size: ½ cup (cooked)

Preparation: Boil steel-cut oats in water or milk until tender, use in breakfast bowls or as a side dish.

Buckwheat Groats

GI Value: 51

GL Value: 16

Portion Size: ½ cup (cooked)

Preparation: Cook buckwheat groats, use in salads, porridge, or as a side dish.

Rye Flakes

GI Value: 34

GL Value: 11

Portion Size: ½ cup (cooked)

Preparation: Cook rye flakes, use in hot cereals, or mix into baked goods.

Sorghum

GI Value: 62

GL Value: 23

Portion Size: ½ cup (cooked)

Preparation: Cook sorghum, use in salads, pilafs, or as a side dish.

Cornmeal (Polenta)

GI Value: 68

GL Value: 20

Portion Size: ½ cup (cooked)

Preparation: Cook cornmeal into polenta, serve as a side dish or use in various recipes.

Bran Flakes Cereal

GI Value: 74

GL Value: 11

Portion Size: ¾ cup

Preparation: Serve bran flakes with milk or yogurt for breakfast.

Buckwheat Flakes Cereal

GI Value: 51

GL Value: 14

Portion Size: ¾ cup

Preparation: Enjoy buckwheat flakes with milk or yogurt as a breakfast cereal.

Whole Grain Puffed Rice Cereal

GI Value: 60

GL Value: 14

Portion Size: 1 cup

Preparation: Have whole grain puffed rice cereal with milk or yogurt for breakfast.

Oat Bran Cereal

GI Value: 50

GL Value: 12

Portion Size: ½ cup

Preparation: Enjoy oat bran cereal with milk or yogurt for breakfast or as a topping

❖ **Proteins and Dairy**

PROTEINS:

Chicken Breast (Skinless, Grilled)

GI Value: 0

GL Value: 0

Portion Size: 3-4 oz (cooked)

Preparation: Marinate chicken with herbs, grill until cooked through, and serve with vegetables.

Turkey Breast (Skinless, Roasted)

GI Value: 0

GL Value: 0

Portion Size: 3-4 oz (cooked)

Preparation: Roast turkey breast with minimal seasoning for a lean protein source.

Salmon Fillet (Grilled or Baked)

GI Value: 0

GL Value: 0

Portion Size: 3-4 oz (cooked)

Preparation: Season salmon with herbs, grill or bake until flaky, and serve with a side of steamed vegetables.

Tofu

GI Value: 15

GL Value: 0

Portion Size: ½ cup (cubed)

Preparation: Press tofu to remove excess water, marinate, and then bake, stir-fry, or grill for various dishes.

Tempeh

GI Value: 35

GL Value: 0

Portion Size: ½ cup (cubed)

Preparation: Marinate tempeh and then bake, grill, or sauté as a meat substitute.

Eggs (Boiled or Poached)

GI Value: 0

GL Value: 0

Portion Size: 2 eggs

Preparation: Boil or poach eggs and enjoy as a breakfast protein or in salads.

Lean Beef (Grilled or Roasted)

GI Value: 0

GL Value: 0

Portion Size: 3-4 oz (cooked)

Preparation: Grill or roast lean cuts of beef and pair with non-starchy vegetables.

Pork Loin (Grilled or Oven-Baked)

GI Value: 0

GL Value: 0

Portion Size: 3-4 oz (cooked)

Preparation: Marinate pork loin with spices, grill, or bake until cooked through.

Lentils

GI Value: 28

GL Value: 5

Portion Size: ½ cup (cooked)

Preparation: Cook lentils and use in soups, salads, or as a side dish.

Chickpeas (Garbanzo Beans)

GI Value: 28

GL Value: 9

Portion Size: ½ cup (cooked)

Preparation: Cook chickpeas and use in salads, curries, or roast for a crunchy snack.

DAIRY:

Greek Yogurt (Plain, Unsweetened)

GI Value: 0

GL Value: 0

Portion Size: 1 cup

Preparation: Enjoy Greek yogurt plain or with fresh fruits and nuts as a snack or breakfast.

Cottage Cheese (Low-fat)

GI Value: 10

GL Value: 3

Portion Size: ½ cup

Preparation: Pair cottage cheese with fruits or use it as a topping for salads.

Skim Milk

GI Value: 32

GL Value: 4

Portion Size: 1 cup

Preparation: Enjoy skim milk as is or use it in smoothies and cereal.

Unsweetened Almond Milk

GI Value: 25

GL Value: 1

Portion Size: 1 cup

Preparation: Use almond milk in smoothies, coffee, or with cereals.

Unflavored Whey Protein Powder

GI Value: Varies

GL Value: Varies

Portion Size: Follow package instructions

Preparation: Mix whey protein powder with water or milk as a post-workout shake or meal replacement.

Low-Fat Mozzarella Cheese

GI Value: 0

GL Value: 0

Portion Size: 1 oz

Preparation: Use mozzarella cheese in salads, sandwiches, or as a topping for pizzas.

Feta Cheese

GI Value: 0

GL Value: 0

Portion Size: 1 oz

Preparation: Crumble feta cheese on salads or use it in Mediterranean-inspired dishes.

Swiss Cheese

GI Value: 0

GL Value: 0

Portion Size: 1 oz

Preparation: Enjoy Swiss cheese as a snack or in sandwiches and wraps.

Plain Kefir

GI Value: 30

GL Value: 4

Portion Size: 1 cup

Preparation: Drink plain kefir or blend it with fruits for a nutritious smoothie.

Ricotta Cheese (Part-Skim)

GI Value: 0

GL Value: 0

Portion Size: ½ cup

Preparation: Use ricotta cheese in pasta dishes, lasagna, or as a spread on toast.

❖ **Legumes**

Lentils

GI Value: 29

GL Value: 5

Portion Size: ½ cup cooked

Preparation: Rinse lentils, cook in water or broth until tender. Use as a side dish or in soups and salads.

Chickpeas (Garbanzo Beans)

GI Value: 28

GL Value: 9

Portion Size: ½ cup cooked

Preparation: Soak dried chickpeas overnight, then boil until tender. Use in curries, hummus, or roast for a crunchy snack.

Black Beans

GI Value: 30

GL Value: 7

Portion Size: ½ cup cooked

Preparation: Soak dried black beans, then cook until soft. Use in salads, soups, or as a filling for tacos or burritos.

Kidney Beans

GI Value: 29

GL Value: 7

Portion Size: ½ cup cooked

Preparation: Soak dried kidney beans, then simmer until cooked. Add to chili, stews, or rice dishes.

Split Peas

GI Value: 25

GL Value: 4

Portion Size: ½ cup cooked

Preparation: Rinse split peas, then simmer until they become mushy. Use in soups or purees.

Lima Beans

GI Value: 32

GL Value: 6

Portion Size: ½ cup cooked

Preparation: Soak dried lima beans, then cook until tender. Use in salads or mixed vegetable dishes.

Cannellini Beans

GI Value: 31

GL Value: 6

Portion Size: ½ cup cooked

Preparation: Soak dried cannellini beans, then cook until soft. Use in pasta dishes or as a side dish.

Pinto Beans

GI Value: 39

GL Value: 9

Portion Size: ½ cup cooked

Preparation: Soak dried pinto beans, then cook until tender. Use in Mexican-inspired dishes or as a side dish.

Adzuki Beans

GI Value: 19

GL Value: 10

Portion Size: ½ cup cooked

Preparation: Soak dried adzuki beans, then cook until soft. Use in sweet or savory dishes.

Mung Beans

GI Value: 25

GL Value: 5

Portion Size: ½ cup cooked

Preparation: Rinse mung beans, then cook until tender. Use in stir-fries or salads.

Black-Eyed Peas

GI Value: 33

GL Value: 10

Portion Size: ½ cup cooked

Preparation: Soak dried black-eyed peas, then cook until soft. Use in soups, stews, or salads.

Fava Beans

GI Value: 33

GL Value: 4

Portion Size: ½ cup cooked

Preparation: Shell fresh fava beans and blanch them. serve as a side dish or in salads.

Great Northern Beans

GI Value: 31

GL Value: 6

Portion Size: ½ cup cooked

Preparation: Soak dried great northern beans, then cook until tender. Use in casseroles or soups.

Navy Beans

GI Value: 38

GL Value: 11

Portion Size: ½ cup cooked

Preparation: Soak dried navy beans, then cook until soft. Use in baked dishes or stews.

Lupini Beans

GI Value: 32

GL Value: 6

Portion Size: ½ cup cooked

Preparation: Soak dried lupini beans in water for several days, changing water daily, then cook until soft. Use as a snack or in salads.

Cowpeas (Black-Eyed Cowpeas)

GI Value: 31

GL Value: 9

Portion Size: ½ cup cooked

Preparation: Soak dried cowpeas, then cook until tender. Use as a side dish or in stews.

Chana Dal (Split Chickpeas)

GI Value: 8

GL Value: 2

Portion Size: ½ cup cooked

Preparation: Rinse chana dal, then cook until soft. Use in Indian dishes or soups.

Lentils (Red)

GI Value: 21

GL Value: 10

Portion Size: ½ cup cooked

Preparation: Rinse red lentils, then cook until they turn mushy. Use in curries or soups.

Yellow Split Peas

GI Value: 25

GL Value: 6

Portion Size: ½ cup cooked

Preparation: Rinse yellow split peas, then cook until soft. Use in soups or purees.

Black Gram (Urad Dal)

GI Value: 30

GL Value: 7

Portion Size: ½ cup cooked

Preparation: Rinse black gram, then cook until soft. Use in Indian cuisine or stews.

❖ **Non-Starchy Vegetables**

Spinach

GI Value: 6

GL Value: 0.2

Portion Size: 1 cup raw or ½ cup cooked

Preparation: Wash spinach thoroughly and use in salads, sautés, or as a side dish.

Broccoli

GI Value: 10

GL Value: 0.4

Portion Size: 1 cup raw or cooked

Preparation: Steam, roast, or stir-fry broccoli as a side dish or add to salads and soups.

Kale

GI Value: 15

GL Value: 0.6

Portion Size: 1 cup raw or cooked

Preparation: Massage kale for salads or lightly sauté with olive oil and garlic.

Cauliflower

GI Value: 15

GL Value: 0.5

Portion Size: 1 cup raw or cooked

Preparation: Roast cauliflower florets, mash as a potato substitute, or use in curries and soups.

Asparagus

GI Value: 15

GL Value: 0.3

Portion Size: 1 cup raw or cooked

Preparation: Grill, steam, or roast asparagus and serve as a side dish or in salads.

Bell Peppers (Green, Red, Yellow)

GI Value: 10

GL Value: 0.4

Portion Size: 1 cup raw or cooked

Preparation: Slice and use raw in salads, stir-fries, or roast as a side dish.

Zucchini

GI Value: 15

GL Value: 0.5

Portion Size: 1 cup raw or cooked

Preparation: Spiralize zucchini for noodles, grill slices, or use in stir-fries and casseroles.

Cabbage

GI Value: 10

GL Value: 0.1

Portion Size: 1 cup raw or cooked

Preparation: Shred for coleslaw, sauté with other vegetables, or use in soups and stews.

Brussels Sprouts

GI Value: 15

GL Value: 0.5

Portion Size: 1 cup raw or cooked

Preparation: Roast, steam, or sauté Brussels sprouts as a side dish or in salads.

Arugula

GI Value: 15

GL Value: 0.2

Portion Size: 1 cup raw

Preparation: Use arugula as a base for salads or add to sandwiches and wraps.

Cucumber

GI Value: 15

GL Value: 0.1

Portion Size: 1 cup raw

Preparation: Slice cucumber for salads, use in sandwiches, or enjoy as a crunchy snack.

Eggplant

GI Value: 15

GL Value: 0.6

Portion Size: 1 cup cooked

Preparation: Roast, grill, or bake eggplant slices for use in casseroles or as a side dish.

Green Beans

GI Value: 15

GL Value: 0.6

Portion Size: 1 cup raw or cooked

Preparation: Steam, sauté, or stir-fry green beans and use as a side dish or in salads.

Onions

GI Value: 10

GL Value: 1

Portion Size: ½ cup raw or cooked

Preparation: Sauté or caramelize onions for use in various dishes, soups, and stews.

Mushrooms

GI Value: 10

GL Value: 0.5

Portion Size: 1 cup raw or cooked

Preparation: Sauté, grill, or roast mushrooms and use in omelets, stir-fries, or as a side dish.

Celery

GI Value: 15

GL Value: 0.5

Portion Size: 1 cup raw

Preparation: Use celery in salads, soups, or enjoy with nut butter as a snack.

Snow Peas

GI Value: 15

GL Value: 0.4

Portion Size: 1 cup raw or cooked

Preparation: Steam, stir-fry, or use snow peas in salads and Asian-inspired dishes.

Artichokes

GI Value: 15

GL Value: 0.4

Portion Size: 1 medium cooked

Preparation: Steam or boil artichokes and serve with a dipping sauce or add to salads.

Leeks

GI Value: 15

GL Value: 0.4

Portion Size: ½ cup raw or cooked

Preparation: Slice and sauté leeks for use in soups, quiches, or as a side dish.

Radishes

GI Value: 15

GL Value: 0.1

Portion Size: 1 cup raw

Preparation: Slice or chop radishes for salads, use in slaws, or enjoy as a crunchy snack.

❖ **Berries**

Strawberries

GI Value: 40

GL Value: 3

Portion Size: 1 cup fresh

Preparation: Rinse and enjoy strawberries whole, sliced in salads, blended in smoothies, or as a topping for yogurt.

Blueberries

GI Value: 53

GL Value: 5

Portion Size: 1 cup fresh

Preparation: Wash blueberries and add them to cereals, oatmeal, yogurt, or use in baking recipes.

Raspberries

GI Value: 32

GL Value: 3

Portion Size: 1 cup fresh

Preparation: Rinse raspberries and use them in salads, desserts, smoothies, or enjoy them on their own.

Blackberries

GI Value: 25

GL Value: 4

Portion Size: 1 cup fresh

Preparation: Wash blackberries and incorporate them into fruit salads, yogurt, or as a topping for pancakes or waffles.

Cranberries

GI Value: 45

GL Value: 5

Portion Size: 1 cup fresh

Preparation: Use fresh cranberries in sauces, chutneys, or bake them into muffins and bread.

Goji Berries

GI Value: 29

GL Value: 4

Portion Size: 1 ounce (about 1/4 cup)

Preparation: Add dried goji berries to trail mix, oatmeal, yogurt, or use them in baked goods.

Acai Berries

GI Value: 11

GL Value: 1

Portion Size: 1 packet or serving

Preparation: Blend frozen acai berries into smoothie bowls, mix with yogurt, or use as a topping.

Cherries

GI Value: 22

GL Value: 3

Portion Size: 1 cup fresh

Preparation: Pit cherries and use them in fruit salads, desserts, or enjoy as a healthy snack.

Strawberry Guavas (Feijoas)

GI Value: 35

GL Value: 4

Portion Size: 1 fruit

Preparation: Slice strawberry guavas and eat them fresh, or use them in fruit salads and smoothies.

Boysenberries

GI Value: 43

GL Value: 4

Portion Size: 1 cup fresh

Preparation: Wash boysenberries and add them to yogurt, oatmeal, or use in baking.

Huckleberries

GI Value: 35

GL Value: 3

Portion Size: 1 cup fresh

Preparation: Enjoy huckleberries fresh, in jams, or as a topping for desserts.

Elderberries

GI Value: 43

GL Value: 4

Portion Size: 1 cup fresh

Preparation: Use elderberries in jams, jellies, syrups, or bake them into pies and tarts.

Loganberries

GI Value: 32

GL Value: 4

Portion Size: 1 cup fresh

Preparation: Wash loganberries and use them in fruit salads, smoothies, or as a topping for ice cream.

Marionberries

GI Value: 35

GL Value: 4

Portion Size: 1 cup fresh

Preparation: Incorporate marionberries into cobblers, jams, or enjoy them fresh.

Mulberries

GI Value: 25

GL Value: 4

Portion Size: 1 cup fresh

Preparation: Use mulberries in fruit salads, smoothies, or bake them into muffins and pies.

Currants (Black, Red, White)

GI Value: 30

GL Value: 3

Portion Size: 1 cup fresh

Preparation: Enjoy currants fresh, in jams, or use them as toppings for desserts.

Cloudberries

GI Value: 25

GL Value: 3

Portion Size: 1 cup fresh

Preparation: Use cloudberries in preserves, jams, or enjoy them fresh with cream or yogurt.

Saskatoon Berries

GI Value: 35

GL Value: 3

Portion Size: 1 cup fresh

Preparation: Enjoy saskatoon berries fresh, in pies, jams, or as a topping for pancakes.

Serviceberries

GI Value: 35

GL Value: 3

Portion Size: 1 cup fresh

Preparation: Use serviceberries in desserts, jams, or enjoy them fresh with yogurt.

Bilberries

GI Value: 25

GL Value: 3

Portion Size: 1 cup fresh

Preparation: Use bilberries in smoothies, bake them into muffins, or enjoy them fresh.

❖ **Quinoa**

White Quinoa

GI Value: 53

GL Value: 13

Portion Size: ½ cup cooked

Preparation: Rinse quinoa, cook in water or broth (1:2 ratio) for 15-20 minutes until fluffy. Use as a base for salads, as a side dish, or in soups.

Red Quinoa

GI Value: 53

GL Value: 13

Portion Size: ½ cup cooked

Preparation: Rinse quinoa, cook in water or broth (1:2 ratio) for 15-20 minutes until tender. Use in pilafs, grain bowls, or as a side dish.

Black Quinoa

GI Value: 53

GL Value: 13

Portion Size: ½ cup cooked

Preparation: Rinse quinoa, cook in water or broth (1:2 ratio) for 15-20 minutes until cooked. Use in salads, stir-fries, or as a base for proteins.

Tri-Color Quinoa (Blend of White, Red, and Black)

GI Value: 53

GL Value: 13

Portion Size: ½ cup cooked

Preparation: Rinse quinoa, cook in water or broth (1:2 ratio) for 15-20 minutes until all water is absorbed. Use in various dishes for added color and texture.

Quinoa Flakes

GI Value: 53

GL Value: 13

Portion Size: ¼ cup dry (equivalent to ½ cup cooked)

Preparation: Cook quinoa flakes in hot water for a few minutes until they thicken. Use as a hot cereal, in baking, or as a substitute for oats.

Sprouted Quinoa

GI Value: 53

GL Value: 13

Portion Size: ½ cup cooked

Preparation: Rinse and soak quinoa until sprouts form, then cook as usual. Use in salads, wraps, or as a base for Buddha bowls.

Organic Quinoa

GI Value: 53

GL Value: 13

Portion Size: ½ cup cooked

Preparation: Rinse organic quinoa thoroughly, cook in water or broth, and use as a versatile base for different dishes.

Instant Quinoa

GI Value: 53

GL Value: 13

Portion Size: Follow package instructions

Preparation: Follow package directions for preparation. Use as a quick side dish or base for meals when time is limited.

Ancient Grains Blend with Quinoa

GI Value: 53

GL Value: 13

Portion Size: ½ cup cooked

Preparation: Cook the blend as per package instructions. Use as a diverse grain base for salads, soups, or as a side dish.

Quinoa Pasta

GI Value: 53

GL Value: 13

Portion Size: Follow package instructions

Preparation: Cook quinoa pasta as directed, use as a gluten-free alternative in pasta dishes.

Quinoa Flour

GI Value: 53

GL Value: 13

Portion Size: Follow recipe instructions

Preparation: Use quinoa flour in baking recipes as a gluten-free option for bread, pancakes, or muffins.

Quinoa Meal

GI Value: 53

GL Value: 13

Portion Size: Follow recipe instructions

Preparation: Cook quinoa meal in water or broth and use as a base for various dishes like casseroles or grain bowls.

Quinoa Bars

GI Value: 53

GL Value: 13

Portion Size: Follow package recommendations

Preparation: Purchase or make quinoa-based bars as a convenient snack option.

Quinoa Cereal

GI Value: 53

GL Value: 13

Portion Size: Follow package instructions

Preparation: Cook quinoa cereal in water or milk, add fruits or nuts for a nutritious breakfast option.

Quinoa Risotto

GI Value: 53

GL Value: 13

Portion Size: ½ cup cooked

Preparation: Prepare quinoa similarly to traditional risotto, using broth and vegetables for a healthy alternative.

Quinoa Salad Mix

GI Value: 53

GL Value: 13

Portion Size: Follow package instructions

Preparation: Use a pre-made mix, typically including quinoa, vegetables, and dressing, as a quick and healthy meal option.

Quinoa Stuffed Peppers

GI Value: 53

GL Value: 13

Portion Size: ½ cup cooked per serving

Preparation: Cook quinoa and use it as a stuffing for bell peppers along with vegetables, herbs, and cheese.

Quinoa Tabbouleh

GI Value: 53

GL Value: 13

Portion Size: ½ cup cooked per serving

Preparation: Mix cooked quinoa with chopped parsley, tomatoes, cucumbers, olive oil, and lemon juice for a refreshing salad.

Quinoa Breakfast Bowl

GI Value: 53

GL Value: 13

Portion Size: ½ cup cooked per serving

Preparation: Combine cooked quinoa with Greek yogurt, fruits, nuts, and honey for a nutritious breakfast bowl.

Quinoa Stir-Fry

GI Value: 53

GL Value: 13

Portion Size: ½ cup cooked per serving

Preparation: Use cooked quinoa in stir-fries with mixed vegetables, tofu or chicken, and soy sauce for a balanced meal.

❖ **Glycemic Steel-Cut Oats Options**

Regular Steel-Cut Oats

GI Value: 55

GL Value: 11

Portion Size: ½ cup uncooked (1 cup cooked)

Preparation: Boil 1 part oats with 3-4 parts water for 20-30 minutes until tender. Serve with toppings like fruits, nuts, or seeds.

Organic Steel-Cut Oats

GI Value: 55

GL Value: 11

Portion Size: ½ cup uncooked (1 cup cooked)

Preparation: Cook organic steel-cut oats in water or milk, adding flavors like cinnamon or vanilla for taste.

Gluten-Free Steel-Cut Oats

GI Value: 55

GL Value: 11

Portion Size: ½ cup uncooked (1 cup cooked)

Preparation: Cook gluten-free steel-cut oats in water or dairy-free milk alternatives for a gluten-free breakfast option.

Irish-Style Steel-Cut Oats

GI Value: 55

GL Value: 11

Portion Size: ½ cup uncooked (1 cup cooked)

Preparation: Simmer Irish-style steel-cut oats in water or milk until creamy. Serve with honey or fresh berries.

Quick Cooking Steel-Cut Oats

GI Value: 55

GL Value: 11

Portion Size: ½ cup uncooked (1 cup cooked)

Preparation: Cook quick-cooking steel-cut oats in boiling water for a shorter time than regular oats. Add fruits or nuts for extra flavor.

Toasted Steel-Cut Oats

GI Value: 55

GL Value: 11

Portion Size: ½ cup uncooked (1 cup cooked)

Preparation: Toast oats lightly in a dry skillet before cooking in water or milk to add a nutty flavor to your breakfast.

Cinnamon Flavored Steel-Cut Oats

GI Value: 55

GL Value: 11

Portion Size: ½ cup uncooked (1 cup cooked)

Preparation: Cook steel-cut oats with cinnamon sticks or ground cinnamon for added flavor without additional sugar.

Apple Cinnamon Steel-Cut Oats

GI Value: 55

GL Value: 11

Portion Size: ½ cup uncooked (1 cup cooked)

Preparation: Cook oats with diced apples and cinnamon for a naturally sweetened breakfast option.

Maple Flavored Steel-Cut Oats

GI Value: 55

GL Value: 11

Portion Size: ½ cup uncooked (1 cup cooked)

Preparation: Add a touch of maple syrup or maple extract while cooking for a hint of sweetness.

Honey Almond Steel-Cut Oats

GI Value: 55

GL Value: 11

Portion Size: ½ cup uncooked (1 cup cooked)

Preparation: Cook oats with almond milk, honey, and sliced almonds for a flavorful, protein-rich breakfast.

Coconut Flavored Steel-Cut Oats

GI Value: 55

GL Value: 11

Portion Size: ½ cup uncooked (1 cup cooked)

Preparation: Use coconut milk instead of water or regular milk for a creamy, tropical twist.

Vanilla Bean Steel-Cut Oats

GI Value: 55

GL Value: 11

Portion Size: ½ cup uncooked (1 cup cooked)

Preparation: Cook oats with a vanilla bean pod or vanilla extract for a fragrant and delightful breakfast.

Pumpkin Spice Steel-Cut Oats

GI Value: 55

GL Value: 11

Portion Size: ½ cup uncooked (1 cup cooked)

Preparation: Add pumpkin puree and spices like cinnamon, nutmeg, and cloves while cooking for a fall-inspired breakfast.

Chocolate Flavored Steel-Cut Oats

GI Value: 55

GL Value: 11

Portion Size: ½ cup uncooked (1 cup cooked)

Preparation: Stir in cocoa powder or dark chocolate chips while cooking for a rich, indulgent morning meal.

Berry-Infused Steel-Cut Oats

GI Value: 55

GL Value: 11

Portion Size: ½ cup uncooked (1 cup cooked)

Preparation: Add fresh or frozen berries (like blueberries, strawberries, or raspberries) while cooking for a fruity breakfast.

Ginger Spiced Steel-Cut Oats

GI Value: 55

GL Value: 11

Portion Size: ½ cup uncooked (1 cup cooked)

Preparation: Incorporate fresh or ground ginger into the cooking process for a warming and flavorful breakfast option.

Chia Seed Steel-Cut Oats

GI Value: 55

GL Value: 11

Portion Size: ½ cup uncooked (1 cup cooked)

Preparation: Add chia seeds while cooking to increase fiber and omega-3 content in your oats.

Nut Butter Steel-Cut Oats

GI Value: 55

GL Value: 11

Portion Size: ½ cup uncooked (1 cup cooked)

Preparation: Stir in a spoonful of peanut butter or almond butter for added creaminess and protein.

Turmeric Spiced Steel-Cut Oats

GI Value: 55

GL Value: 11

Portion Size: ½ cup uncooked (1 cup cooked)

Preparation: Incorporate turmeric powder while cooking for its anti-inflammatory properties and unique flavor.

Lemon Blueberry Steel-Cut Oats

GI Value: 55

GL Value: 11

Portion Size: ½ cup uncooked (1 cup cooked)

Preparation: Add lemon zest and fresh blueberries during cooking for a refreshing and tangy breakfast option.

❖ **Nuts:**

Walnuts

GI Value: 15

GL Value: 1

Portion Size: 1 ounce (about 14 halves)

Preparation: Enjoy walnuts raw as a snack, in salads, or as a topping for yogurt or oatmeal.

Almonds

GI Value: 0

GL Value: 0

Portion Size: 1 ounce (about 23 almonds)

Preparation: Eat almonds raw as a snack or add them to trail mix or homemade granola.

Pistachios

GI Value: 14

GL Value: 1

Portion Size: 1 ounce (about 49 kernels)

Preparation: Enjoy pistachios as a snack or sprinkle them over salads or yogurt.

Cashews

GI Value: 25

GL Value: 5

Portion Size: 1 ounce (about 18 nuts)

Preparation: Eat cashews raw or roasted, add them to stir-fries, or use them in nut butter.

Hazelnuts

GI Value: 0

GL Value: 0

Portion Size: 1 ounce (about 21 nuts)

Preparation: Enjoy hazelnuts raw, roasted, or as part of baked goods and desserts.

Brazil Nuts

GI Value: 11

GL Value: 0

Portion Size: 1 ounce (about 6 nuts)

Preparation: Eat Brazil nuts raw or chop and add them to salads or oatmeal.

Pecans

GI Value: 0

GL Value: 0

Portion Size: 1 ounce (about 19 halves)

Preparation: Enjoy pecans raw as a snack or use them in baking and cooking.

Macadamia Nuts

GI Value: 0

GL Value: 0

Portion Size: 1 ounce (about 10-12 nuts)

Preparation: Eat macadamia nuts raw or use them in cookies, granola, or salads.

Pine Nuts

GI Value: 15

GL Value: 0

Portion Size: 1 ounce (about 167 kernels)

Preparation: Enjoy pine nuts in pesto, salads, or as a topping for dishes.

Chia Seeds

GI Value: 1

GL Value: 0

Portion Size: 1 ounce (about 2 tablespoons)

Preparation: Mix chia seeds into yogurt, smoothies, or use them as an egg substitute in baking.

Flaxseeds

GI Value: 1

GL Value: 0

Portion Size: 1 ounce (about 2 tablespoons)

Preparation: Ground flaxseeds and add them to smoothies, oatmeal, or use as an egg substitute.

Sunflower Seeds

GI Value: 10

GL Value: 1

Portion Size: 1 ounce (about 2 tablespoons)

Preparation: Enjoy sunflower seeds raw or roasted, add them to salads or baked goods.

Hemp Seeds

GI Value: 0

GL Value: 0

Portion Size: 1 ounce (about 2 tablespoons)

Preparation: Sprinkle hemp seeds on salads, yogurt, or blend into smoothies.

Sesame Seeds

GI Value: 0

GL Value: 0

Portion Size: 1 ounce (about 3 tablespoons)

Preparation: Toast sesame seeds and use them in stir-fries, salads, or as a seasoning.

Pumpkin Seeds (Pepitas)

GI Value: 15

GL Value: 1

Portion Size: 1 ounce (about 85 seeds)

Preparation: Enjoy pumpkin seeds raw or roasted, add them to salads or granola.

Poppy Seeds

GI Value: 0

GL Value: 0

Portion Size: 1 ounce (about 3 tablespoons)

Preparation: Use poppy seeds in baking, salad dressings, or as a topping for bread.

Quinoa

GI Value: 53

GL Value: 13

Portion Size: 1 ounce (about 2 tablespoons)

Preparation: Rinse quinoa and cook it as a side dish or use it in salads and soups.

Amaranth

GI Value: 46

GL Value: 11

Portion Size: 1 ounce (about 3 tablespoons)

Preparation: Cook amaranth and use it in porridge, salads, or baked goods.

Buckwheat Groats

GI Value: 51

GL Value: 16

Portion Size: 1 ounce (about 3 tablespoons)

Preparation: Cook buckwheat groats and use them in pilafs, salads, or as a side dish.

Brown Rice

GI Value: 50

GL Value: 16

Portion Size: 1 ounce (about 2 tablespoons)

Preparation: Cook brown rice and use it in various dishes such as stir-fries or salads.

❖ **Leafy Greens:**

Spinach

GI Value: 15

GL Value: 0

Portion Size: 1 cup (raw)

Preparation: Use spinach in salads, sandwiches, or sauté lightly as a side dish.

Kale

GI Value: 15

GL Value: 1

Portion Size: 1 cup (raw)

Preparation: Massage kale for salads, bake as kale chips, or add to soups and smoothies.

Swiss Chard

GI Value: 15

GL Value: 1

Portion Size: 1 cup (cooked)

Preparation: Sauté Swiss chard with garlic, add to omelets, or use in stir-fries.

Collard Greens

GI Value: 10

GL Value: 0

Portion Size: 1 cup (cooked)

Preparation: Boil or steam collard greens, use as wraps, or in soups and stews.

Arugula

GI Value: 15

GL Value: 0

Portion Size: 1 cup (raw)

Preparation: Use arugula in salads, as a pizza topping, or blend into pesto.

Romaine Lettuce

GI Value: 15

GL Value: 0

Portion Size: 1 cup (raw)

Preparation: Use romaine lettuce in salads, wraps, or as a bed for various dishes.

Bok Choy

GI Value: 10

GL Value: 0

Portion Size: 1 cup (cooked)

Preparation: Stir-fry bok choy with garlic and ginger or add to soups and Asian dishes.

Watercress

GI Value: 15

GL Value: 0

Portion Size: 1 cup (raw)

Preparation: Use watercress in salads, sandwiches, or blend into soups.

Beet Greens

GI Value: 15

GL Value: 0

Portion Size: 1 cup (cooked)

Preparation: Sauté beet greens with olive oil and garlic or add them to stews.

Dandelion Greens

GI Value: 15

GL Value: 0

Portion Size: 1 cup (raw)

Preparation: Use dandelion greens in salads, smoothies, or sauté with onions and herbs.

Mustard Greens

GI Value: 15

GL Value: 0

Portion Size: 1 cup (cooked)

Preparation: Cook mustard greens in soups, stir-fries, or sauté with spices.

Turnip Greens

GI Value: 15

GL Value: 0

Portion Size: 1 cup (cooked)

Preparation: Cook turnip greens and use them in casseroles, soups, or as a side dish.

Microgreens (Various Types)

GI Value: Varies (Generally low)

GL Value: Varies

Portion Size: Varies by type (usually a handful)

Preparation: Use microgreens in salads, sandwiches, or as garnishes for various dishes.

Cabbage (Green or Red)

GI Value: 10

GL Value: 0

Portion Size: 1 cup (raw)

Preparation: Use cabbage in salads, coleslaw, stir-fries, or ferment for sauerkraut.

Iceberg Lettuce

GI Value: 15

GL Value: 0

Portion Size: 1 cup (raw)

Preparation: Use iceberg lettuce in salads, sandwiches, or as a bed for dishes.

Endive

GI Value: 15

GL Value: 0

Portion Size: 1 cup (raw)

Preparation: Use endive in salads, as a garnish, or fill leaves with various fillings.

Cilantro (Coriander Leaves)

GI Value: 15

GL Value: 0

Portion Size: 1 cup (raw)

Preparation: Use cilantro in salads, salsas, sauces, or as a garnish.

Parsley

GI Value: 15

GL Value: 0

Portion Size: 1 cup (raw)

Preparation: Use parsley in salads, as a seasoning, or blend into pesto.

Spring Mix

GI Value: 15

GL Value: 0

Portion Size: 1 cup (raw)

Preparation: Enjoy spring mix in salads, sandwiches, or as a bed for various dishes.

Herbs (Basil, Mint, etc.)

GI Value: Varies (Generally low)

GL Value: Varies

Portion Size: Varies (usually a handful)

Preparation: Use fresh herbs as seasonings, in salads, dressings, or to flavor dishes.

Diabetes management often involves controlling blood sugar levels, and the glycemic index plays a pivotal role in this journey. The glycemic index calculates the rate at which food carbs elevate blood sugar. Low GI foods, with their slower digestion and absorption rates, can help maintain steadier blood sugar levels and are therefore valuable for individuals managing diabetes.

Role of Low GI Foods in Diabetes Management

Low GI foods, typically with values under 55, are known to release glucose more gradually into the bloodstream, preventing spikes in blood sugar levels. These foods offer sustained energy, reduce hunger pangs, and aid in better blood sugar control, key factors for diabetes management. They include whole grains, legumes, non-starchy vegetables, certain fruits, and lean proteins.

Creating Balanced Meals for Diabetes Control

Designing balanced meals involves combining low GI foods with lean proteins and healthy fats. For instance, incorporating whole grains like quinoa or brown rice, paired with vegetables such as leafy greens, broccoli, or bell peppers, forms a solid foundation for a low GI meal. Add in lean proteins like chicken, fish, or tofu and healthy fats from sources like avocados or nuts for a well-rounded, blood sugar-friendly plate.

Tips for Incorporating Low GI Foods into Daily Routine

Educate Yourself: Learn about the GI values of various foods. Opt for whole, unprocessed foods that are naturally low in GI.

Plan Meals: Prepare a weekly meal plan incorporating low GI foods. This helps maintain consistency and reduces impulsive food choices.

Choose low GI snacks like nuts, Greek yogurt, or fruits like apples or berries to maintain blood **Snack Smart:** sugar levels between meals.

Cook Wisely: Experiment with cooking methods. Steaming, baking, or sautéing vegetables and opting for whole grains instead of refined ones can lower the overall GI of meals.

Read Labels: Check food labels for hidden sugars and refined carbohydrates. Pay attention to portion sizes to maintain glycemic control.

Combine Foods: Pair high GI foods with low GI options to moderate their overall impact on blood sugar. For instance, have brown rice with vegetables and protein.

By adopting a low GI diet, individuals with diabetes can better manage blood sugar levels, reduce insulin resistance, and lower the risk of complications associated with the condition.

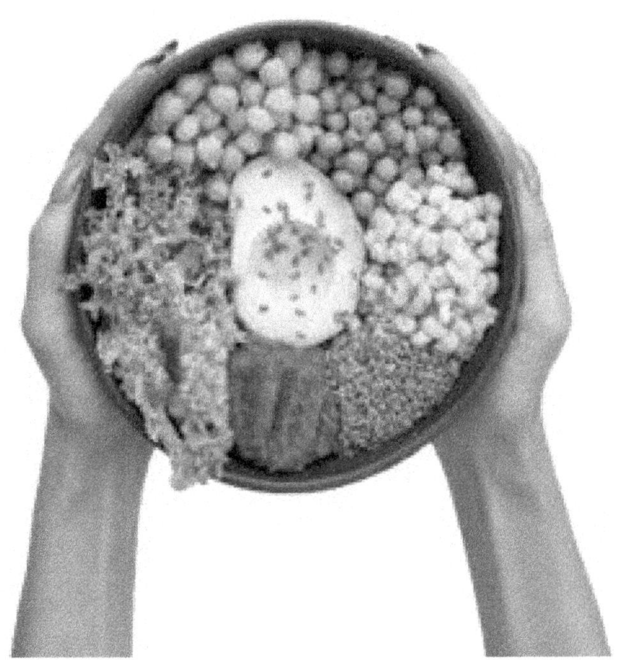

❖ **Breakfast Recipes**

1. Greek Yogurt Parfait

Ingredients:

- 1/2 cup Greek yogurt (unsweetened)
- 1/4 cup mixed berries (strawberries, blueberries, raspberries)
- 1 tablespoon chopped nuts (almonds, walnuts)
- 1 teaspoon honey or a sprinkle of cinnamon (optional)

Preparation:

1. Arrange the Greek yogurt in a bottom layer in a glass or bowl.
2. Top the yogurt with a layer of mixed berries.
3. Sprinkle chopped nuts over the berries.
4. Optionally, drizzle honey for sweetness or sprinkle cinnamon for flavor.
5. Repeat layers if desired.

Portion Size: One serving (adjust ingredient amounts as needed).

Nutritional Information (approx.):

- o Calories: 180-200
- o Protein: 15-20g
- o Carbohydrates: 15-20g
- o Fiber: 3-5g
- o Fat: 7-10g

2. Veggie Omelette

Ingredients:

- 2 eggs
- 1/4 cup diced bell peppers (any color)
- 1/4 cup chopped spinach
- 1 tablespoon chopped onions
- 1 tablespoon olive oil
- Salt and pepper to taste

Preparation:

1. Add salt and pepper to a bowl of whisked eggs.
2. In a nonstick pan, warm the olive oil over medium heat.
3. Sauté onions, bell peppers, and spinach until slightly tender.
4. Pour the whisked eggs over the veggies in the pan.
5. Cook until the omelette is set and edges start to brown.
6. Cut the omelette in half, then warm it through.

Portion Size: One omelette.

Nutritional Information (approx.):

- Calories: 250-300
- Protein: 15-18g
- Carbohydrates: 5-8g
- Fiber: 2-3g
- Fat: 18-22g

3. Overnight Chia Seed Pudding

Ingredients:

- 2 tablespoons chia seeds
- 1/2 cup unsweetened almond milk (or any milk of choice)
- 1/4 teaspoon vanilla extract
- 1 teaspoon honey or a few drops of stevia (optional)
- Sliced fruits (berries, banana) for topping

Preparation:

1. In a bowl or jar, mix chia seeds, almond milk, vanilla extract, and sweetener (if using).
2. Stir well and refrigerate overnight or for at least 4 hours.
3. Before serving, stir the mixture again and top with sliced fruits.

Portion Size: One serving.

Nutritional Information (approx.):

- Calories: 150-180
- Protein: 4-6g

o   Carbohydrates: 12-15g

o   Fiber: 8-10g

o   Fat: 8-10

4. Quinoa Breakfast Bowl

Ingredients:

- 1/2 cup cooked quinoa

- 1/4 cup Greek yogurt

- 1 tablespoon chopped nuts (almonds, pecans)

- 1/4 cup diced apple or pear

- 1 teaspoon honey or a sprinkle of cinnamon (optional)

Preparation:

1. In a bowl, place cooked quinoa as the base.
2. Top the quinoa with a dollop of Greek yogurt.
3. Sprinkle chopped nuts and diced fruits over the yogurt.
4. Optionally, drizzle honey or sprinkle cinnamon for sweetness.

Portion Size: One serving.

Nutritional Information (approx.):

- o   Calories: 250-300
- o   Protein: 10-12g
- o   Carbohydrates: 30-35g
- o   Fiber: 4-6g
- o   Fat: 10-12g

5. Avocado Toast with Egg

Ingredients:

- 1 slice whole-grain bread
- 1/2 ripe avocado
- 1 egg
- Salt, pepper, and red pepper flakes (optional)

Preparation:

1. Toast the whole-grain bread until golden brown.
2. Spread the avocado on the toast after mashing it.
3. Cook the egg (poached, fried, or scrambled) and place it on top of the avocado.
4. If desired, add red pepper flakes, salt, and pepper for seasoning.

Portion Size: One serving.

Nutritional Information (approx.):

- o   Calories: 250-300
- o   Protein: 10-12g
- o   Carbohydrates: 20-25g
- o   Fiber: 6-8g
- o   Fat: 12-15g

1. Grilled Chicken Salad

Ingredients:

- 4 ounces grilled chicken breast (sliced)
- 2 cups mixed greens (spinach, arugula, lettuce)
- 1/4 cup cherry tomatoes (halved)
- 1/4 cucumber (sliced)
- 1/4 avocado (sliced)
- 1 tablespoon olive oil
- 1 tablespoon balsamic vinegar
- Salt and pepper to taste

Preparation:

1. Season grilled chicken with salt and pepper, then slice it.
2. In a large bowl, toss mixed greens, cherry tomatoes, cucumber, and avocado slices.
3. Add grilled chicken slices on top of the salad.
4. Drizzle olive oil and balsamic vinegar as dressing.
5. Toss gently to combine and serve.

Portion Size: One serving.

Nutritional Information (approx.):

- o   Calories: 300-350

- o   Protein: 25-30g

- o   Carbohydrates: 10-12g

- o   Fiber: 5-7g

- o   Fat: 15-18g

2. Lentil Soup

Ingredients:

- 1 cup dried lentils

- 4 cups vegetable or chicken broth

- 1 onion (diced)

- 2 carrots (diced)

- 2 celery stalks (diced)

- 2 cloves garlic (minced)

- 1 teaspoon olive oil

- Salt, pepper, and herbs (such as thyme or rosemary) to taste

Preparation:

1. Rinse lentils thoroughly and set aside.
2. In a pot, heat olive oil over medium heat, add onions, carrots, celery, and garlic. Sauté until vegetables soften.
3. Add lentils and broth to the pot. Season with salt, pepper, and herbs.
4. Bring to a boil, then reduce heat and simmer for about 30-40 minutes until lentils are tender.
5. Adjust seasoning if needed and serve hot.

Portion Size: One serving.

Nutritional Information (approx.):

o Calories: 250-300
o Protein: 15-18g
o Carbohydrates: 40-45g
o Fiber: 15-18g
o Fat: 3-5g

3. Turkey and Veggie Wrap

Ingredients:

- 1 whole-grain tortilla or wrap
- 3 ounces cooked turkey breast slices
- 1/4 cup hummus
- 1/4 cup shredded lettuce
- 1/4 cup sliced bell peppers
- 1/4 cup grated carrots
- 1 tablespoon Greek yogurt (optional)
- Fresh herbs (parsley, cilantro) for flavor

Preparation:

1. Spread hummus evenly on the tortilla.
2. Layer turkey slices, shredded lettuce, bell peppers, and grated carrots on the tortilla.
3. Optionally, add a dollop of Greek yogurt and sprinkle fresh herbs for extra flavor.
4. Roll the tortilla tightly into a wrap and cut in half if desired.

Portion Size: One wrap.

Nutritional Information (approx.):

- o Calories: 300-350
- o Protein: 20-25g
- o Carbohydrates: 25-30g
- o Fiber: 5-8g
- o Fat: 12-15g

4. Quinoa and Vegetable Stir-Fry

Ingredients:

- 1/2 cup cooked quinoa
- 1 cup mixed vegetables (broccoli, bell peppers, snap peas)
- 1 tablespoon low-sodium soy sauce
- 1 teaspoon sesame oil
- 1 garlic clove (minced)
- 1/2 teaspoon grated ginger
- 1 tablespoon olive oil
- Salt and pepper to taste

Preparation:

1. In a pan or wok, heat the olive oil over medium-high heat.
2. Add minced garlic and grated ginger, sauté for a minute.
3. Stir in mixed vegetables and cook until tender-crisp.
4. Add cooked quinoa to the vegetables.
5. Drizzle soy sauce and sesame oil, toss everything together.
6. Season with salt and pepper, then serve hot.

Portion Size: One serving.

Nutritional Information (approx.):

- Calories: 300-350
- Protein: 10-12g
- Carbohydrates: 35-40g
- Fiber: 6-8g
- Fat: 12-15g

5. Baked Salmon with Roasted Vegetables

Ingredients:

- 4 ounces salmon fillet
- 1 cup mixed roasted vegetables (zucchini, eggplant, cherry tomatoes)
- 1 tablespoon olive oil
- Lemon wedges for garnish
- Salt, pepper, and herbs (dill, parsley) for seasoning

Preparation:

1. Preheat oven to 400°F (200°C).
2. Place salmon on a baking sheet, drizzle with olive oil, and season with salt, pepper, and herbs.
3. Arrange mixed vegetables around the salmon on the baking sheet.
4. Bake for 15-20 minutes until salmon is cooked through and vegetables are tender.
5. Serve hot with lemon wedges for garnish.

Portion Size: One serving.

Nutritional Information (approx.):

Calories: 300-350

Protein: 25-30g

Carbohydrates: 10-12g

Fiber: 3-5g

Fat: 18-20g

1. Baked Lemon Herb Chicken

Ingredients:

- 4 skinless, boneless chicken breasts
- 2 tablespoons olive oil
- Juice of 1 lemon
- 2 garlic cloves (minced)
- 1 teaspoon dried thyme
- 1 teaspoon dried rosemary
- Salt and pepper to taste
- Lemon slices for garnish

Preparation:

1. Preheat oven to 375°F (190°C).
2. Place chicken breasts in a baking dish.
3. In a bowl, mix olive oil, lemon juice, minced garlic, thyme, rosemary, salt, and pepper.
4. Pour the mixture over the chicken breasts, ensuring they are coated evenly.

5. Bake the chicken for 25 to 30 minutes, or until it is thoroughly cooked.

6. Garnish with lemon slices before serving.

Portion Size: One chicken breast.

Nutritional Information (approx.):

o   Calories: 200-250

o   Protein: 25-30g

o   Carbohydrates: 0g

o   Fiber: 0g

o   Fat: 10-12g

2. Cauliflower Rice Stir-Fry

Ingredients:

- 1 head cauliflower

- 1 tablespoon sesame oil

- 1 cup mixed vegetables (bell peppers, broccoli, carrots)

- 2 eggs (optional)

- 2 tablespoons low-sodium soy sauce

- 1 teaspoon grated ginger

- 2 garlic cloves (minced)

- Salt and pepper to taste

- Green onions for garnish

Preparation:

1. Grate cauliflower florets into rice-like grains using a grater or food processor.
2. In a pan or wok, warm the sesame oil over medium-high heat.
3. Add the grated ginger and minced garlic and sauté until aromatic.
4. Add mixed vegetables and cauliflower rice to the pan, stir-fry until tender.
5. Optionally, push the rice and vegetables to the side of the pan and scramble eggs on the other side.
6. Combine everything, drizzle soy sauce, and season with salt and pepper.
7. Add chopped green onions as a garnish and serve hot.

Portion Size: One serving.

Nutritional Information (approx.):

- o Calories: 200-250
- o Protein: 8-10g
- o Carbohydrates: 20-25g
- o Fiber: 8-10g
- o Fat: 10-12g

3. Grilled Salmon with Asparagus

Ingredients:

- 4 ounces salmon fillet
- 1/2 bunch asparagus
- 1 tablespoon olive oil
- Lemon wedges for garnish
- Salt, pepper, and herbs (such as dill or parsley) for seasoning

Preparation:

1. Turn the heat up to medium-high on the grill or grill pan.
2. Rub salmon with olive oil and season with salt, pepper, and herbs.
3. Place salmon and asparagus on the grill.

4. Cook the salmon on the grill for 4–5 minutes on each side, or until it is done.

5. Grill asparagus for 3-4 minutes until slightly charred and tender.

6. Serve hot with lemon wedges for garnish.

Portion Size: One serving.

Nutritional Information (approx.):

- o Calories: 250-300
- o Protein: 25-30g
- o Carbohydrates: 5-8g
- o Fiber: 3-5g
- o Fat: 15-18g

4. Turkey and Vegetable Skewers

Ingredients:

- 8 ounces turkey breast, cut into chunks
- 1 bell pepper (cut into chunks)
- 1 zucchini (sliced)
- 1 red onion (cut into chunks)
- 2 tablespoons olive oil
- 1 teaspoon paprika

- 1 teaspoon cumin
- Salt and pepper to taste
- Skewers

Preparation:

1. Turn the heat up to medium-high on the grill or grill pan.
2. In a bowl, toss turkey, bell pepper, zucchini, and red onion with olive oil, paprika, cumin, salt, and pepper.
3. Thread the marinated turkey and vegetables onto skewers.
4. Grill skewers for about 8-10 minutes, turning occasionally until turkey is cooked and veggies are tender.
5. Serve hot.

Portion Size: Two skewers.

Nutritional Information (approx.):

- Calories: 250-300
- Protein: 25-30g
- Carbohydrates: 8-10g
- Fiber: 2-4g

o   Fat: 12-15g

5. Eggplant and Tomato Bake

Ingredients:

- 1 large eggplant (sliced)
- 2 tomatoes (sliced)
- 2 garlic cloves (minced)
- 2 tablespoons olive oil
- 1/4 cup grated Parmesan cheese
- Fresh basil leaves for garnish
- Salt and pepper to taste

Preparation:

1. Preheat oven to 375°F (190°C).
2. Grease a baking dish with olive oil.
3. Arrange slices of eggplant and tomato in layers in the baking dish.
4. Sprinkle minced garlic, salt, and pepper between the layers.
5. Drizzle olive oil over the top layer and sprinkle with grated Parmesan cheese.

6. Bake for 30-35 minutes until vegetables are tender and golden brown.

7. Garnish with fresh basil leaves before serving.

Portion Size: One serving.

Nutritional Information (approx.):

o Calories: 200-250

o Protein: 5-8g

o Carbohydrates: 15-20g

o Fiber: 8-10g

o Fat: 12-15g

1. Apple and Almond Butter Sandwich

Ingredients:

- 1 apple (sliced)
- 2 tablespoons almond butter (unsweetened)

Preparation:

1. Slice the apple into thin rounds.
2. Spread almond butter on half of the apple slices.
3. To make "sandwiches," top with the remaining apple slices.

Portion Size: One apple with almond butter.

Nutritional Information (approx.):

- o Calories: 200-250
- o Protein: 4-6g
- o Carbohydrates: 20-25g
- o Fiber: 5-7g
- o Fat: 12-15g

2. Greek Yogurt with Berries and Nuts

Ingredients:

- 1/2 cup Greek yogurt (unsweetened)
- 1/4 cup mixed berries (blueberries, raspberries)
- 1 tablespoon chopped nuts (almonds, walnuts)

Preparation:

1. Place Greek yogurt in a bowl.
2. Top with mixed berries and chopped nuts.

Portion Size: One serving.

Nutritional Information (approx.):

- Calories: 150-180
- Protein: 12-15g
- Carbohydrates: 10-12g
- Fiber: 2-3g
- Fat: 8-10g

3. Veggie Sticks with Hummus

Ingredients:

- Carrot sticks
- Celery sticks
- Cucumber sticks
- 1/4 cup hummus (unsweetened)

Preparation:

1. Wash and cut vegetables into sticks.
2. Present with a hummus side dish for dipping.

Portion Size: One serving of veggies with hummus.

Nutritional Information (approx.):

- Calories: 100-120
- Protein: 3-5g
- Carbohydrates: 10-12g
- Fiber: 3-5g
- Fat: 5-8g

4. Hard-Boiled Eggs with Avocado

Ingredients:

- 2 hard-boiled eggs
- 1/2 ripe avocado

Preparation:

1. Slice hard-boiled eggs in half.
2. Remove the pit from the avocado and scoop out half.
3. Serve eggs with avocado slices.

Portion Size: Two eggs with half an avocado.

Nutritional Information (approx.):

o Calories: 250-300

o Protein: 15-18g

o Carbohydrates: 8-10g

o Fiber: 6-8g

o Fat: 18-20g

5. Cottage Cheese and Pineapple Bowl

Ingredients:

- 1/2 cup cottage cheese (unsweetened)
- 1/2 cup pineapple chunks (fresh or canned in juice)

Preparation:

1. Place cottage cheese in a bowl.
2. Top with pineapple chunks.

Portion Size: One serving.

Nutritional Information (approx.):

- Calories: 150-180
- Protein: 12-15g
- Carbohydrates: 15-18g
- Fiber: 1-3g
- Fat: 5-8g

❖ **7-Day Meal Plan**

DAY 1:

Breakfast: Greek Yogurt Parfait

Lunch: Lentil Soup

Dinner: Baked Lemon Herb Chicken

Snack: Veggie Sticks with Hummus

DAY 2:

Breakfast: Overnight Chia Seed Pudding

Lunch: Turkey and Vegetable Skewers

Dinner: Quinoa and Vegetable Stir-Fry

Snack: Apple and Almond Butter Sandwich

Breakfast: Veggie Omelette

Lunch: Grilled Chicken Salad

Dinner: Eggplant and Tomato Bake

Snack: Greek Yogurt with Berries and Nuts

DAY 4:

Breakfast: Avocado Toast with Egg

Lunch: Cauliflower Rice Stir-Fry

Dinner: Grilled Salmon with Asparagus

Snack: Cottage Cheese and Pineapple Bowl

DAY 5:

Breakfast: Quinoa Breakfast Bowl

Lunch: Lentil Soup

Dinner: Baked Lemon Herb Chicken

Snack: Veggie Sticks with Hummus

Breakfast: Greek Yogurt Parfait

Lunch: Turkey and Vegetable Skewers

Dinner: Quinoa and Vegetable Stir-Fry

Snack: Apple and Almond Butter Sandwich

Breakfast: Overnight Chia Seed Pudding

Lunch: Grilled Chicken Salad

Dinner: Eggplant and Tomato Bake

Snack: Greek Yogurt with Berries and Nuts

Batch Cooking: Prepare large quantities of staple foods like quinoa, brown rice, or grilled chicken at the start of the week. Use them as the foundation for different meals all week long.

Chop Veggies in Advance: Chop vegetables like bell peppers, carrots, and cucumbers in advance and store them in airtight containers in the fridge. This saves time during meal preparation.

Portion Control: Use portion-sized containers to pre-portion meals for the week, especially for snacks like cottage cheese with pineapple or veggie sticks with hummus.

Make Overnight Preps: Overnight chia seed puddings, yogurt parfaits, or marinating proteins in advance can save time in the morning and add convenience to breakfast and lunch options.

Freeze Smoothie Ingredients: Pre-pack and freeze ingredients for smoothies in individual bags. Simply blend with a liquid base in the morning for a quick and nutritious breakfast.

Prepare Salad Ingredients Separately: If planning salads, keep wet ingredients like tomatoes separate from dry ingredients like lettuce until just before eating to maintain freshness.

Cook Once, Use Twice: When making dinner, cook extra portions for lunch the next day. For instance, baked chicken for dinner can become a chicken salad for lunch.

Utilize Slow Cookers or Instant Pots: Use these appliances to cook soups, stews, or whole grains while you attend to other tasks. They make meal prep quick and hassle-free.

Label and Date: When meal prepping, label containers with the date of preparation to keep track of freshness.

Stay Organized: Plan your meals for the week, create shopping lists based on these plans, and set aside specific prep time to streamline the process.

These meal prep tips can make it easier to stick to a low glycemic index diet, save time during busy days, and ensure you have healthy and balanced meals readily available. Adjust these tips to suit your preferences and lifestyle for optimal success!

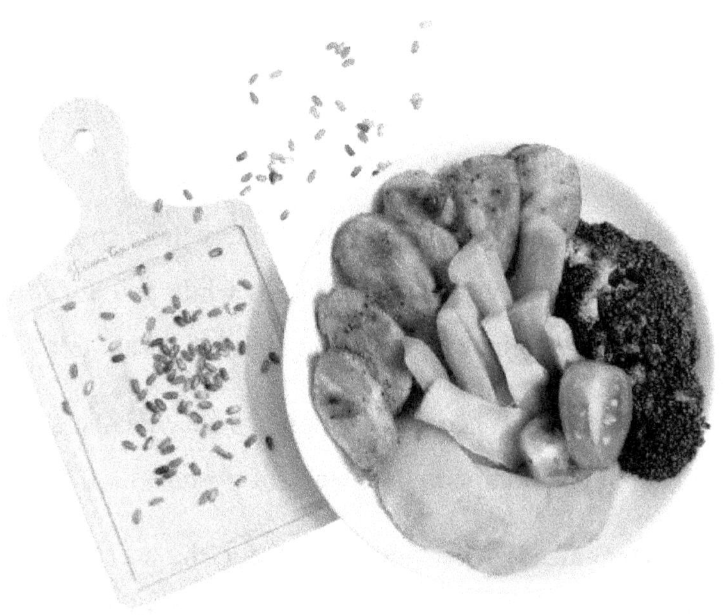

❖ Weight Management with Low GI Foods

Low GI foods help manage weight by regulating blood sugar levels and promoting satiety. These foods provide a slower and more sustained release of energy, reducing cravings and the likelihood of overeating. By stabilizing blood sugar, they assist in weight control and fat loss.

❖ Energy Levels and Sustained Nutrition:

Consuming low GI foods maintains steady blood sugar levels, providing a consistent and prolonged source of energy. This sustained energy helps avoid energy crashes often associated with high GI foods. It aids in improved concentration, endurance during physical activities, and promotes a more balanced mood throughout the day.

❖ **Long-Term Health Benefits:**

Blood Sugar Regulation: Low GI diets support better blood sugar control, crucial for individuals managing diabetes. They help prevent spikes and crashes in blood glucose levels, reducing the risk of insulin resistance and type 2 diabetes.

Heart Health: These diets are associated with better heart health due to their ability to improve lipid profiles. They can lower the risk of cardiovascular diseases and LDL cholesterol levels.

Improved Digestion: High-fiber, low GI foods support digestive health by regulating bowel movements and promoting a healthy gut microbiome.

Reduced Risk of Chronic Diseases: Low GI diets have been linked to a lower risk of certain cancers, particularly those affecting the colon and digestive system. Additionally, they may reduce the risk of developing metabolic syndrome.

Sustained Weight Loss and Maintenance: These diets facilitate sustainable weight loss and assist in weight maintenance by promoting a feeling of fullness and reducing cravings.

Enhanced Longevity: A diet rich in low GI foods has been associated with a longer and healthier lifespan, possibly due to reduced risks of chronic diseases.

Adopting a diet focused on low GI foods can significantly impact overall health and well-being. By incorporating these foods into your daily meals, you can experience sustained energy levels, better weight management, and a reduced risk of chronic illnesses, leading to a healthier and more fulfilling lifestyle.

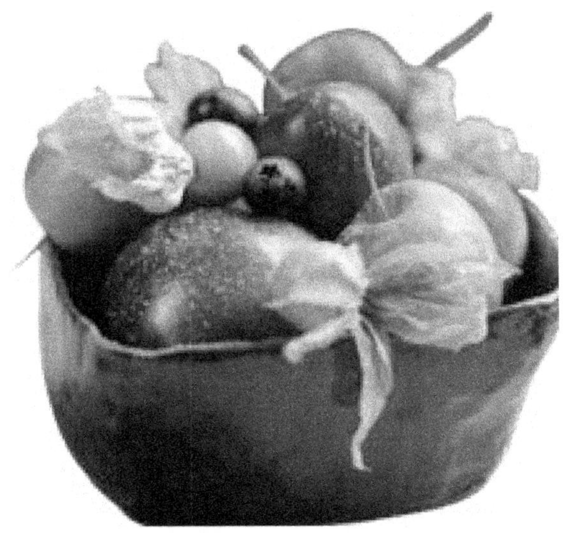

CONCLUSION

As we conclude this insightful journey through the realm of low glycemic index (GI) foods, it becomes evident that this isn't just a guidebook, it's a gateway to a transformed way of nourishing both body and spirit.

Within these pages, we've uncovered the profound impact of choosing foods that gently influence our blood sugar levels, transcending the mere act of eating to embody a philosophy, a philosophy rooted in nurturing our bodies with wisdom and intention.

This book isn't just about recipes and meal plans; it's a manifesto of empowerment, a testament to the incredible potential we hold to sculpt our health through the choices we make daily. It's

about embracing a lifestyle that champions sustained energy, optimal health, and the fortification of our well-being against the tides of chronic ailments.

In its essence, this book isn't merely a compendium of low GI foods; it's an invitation, a call to embark on a transformative journey towards a healthier, more vibrant life. It's an embrace of the myriad benefits that extend beyond the physical, a bolstering of our vitality, a safeguarding of our future, and a celebration of the intricate dance between nutrition and well-being.

May these insights and recipes serve as beacons guiding your culinary adventures, empowering you to curate meals that not only nourish but elevate, a journey where each bite embodies a symphony of health, each recipe a testament to the art of mindful, purposeful eating.

As you close this chapter, may the lessons learned linger, a reminder that the choices on our plates are the brushstrokes that paint the canvas of our wellness. Let this book be a companion on your voyage towards a healthier, more vibrant you, a compass pointing to the transformative power of embracing low GI foods as a cornerstone of a balanced, nourished life.

WEEKLY MEAL PLANNER JOURNAL

WEEK _______________   MONTH _______________

MONDAY

TUESDAY

WEDNESDAY

THURSDAY

FRIDAY

SATURDAY

SUNDAY

SHOPPING LIST

- ○ _______________
- ○ _______________
- ○ _______________
- ○ _______________
- ○ _______________
- ○ _______________
- ○ _______________
- ○ _______________

NOTES:

- ○ _______________
- ○ _______________
- ○ _______________
- ○ _______________

WEEKLY MEAL PLANNER JOURNAL

WEEK _______________   MONTH _______________

MONDAY

SATURDAY

TUESDAY

SUNDAY

WEDNESDAY

SHOPPING LIST

THURSDAY

FRIDAY

NOTES:

WEEKLY MEAL PLANNER JOURNAL

WEEK ___________________   MONTH ___________________

MONDAY

TUESDAY

WEDNESDAY

THURSDAY

FRIDAY

SATURDAY

SUNDAY

SHOPPING LIST

NOTES:

WEEKLY MEAL PLANNER JOURNAL

WEEK ___________________   MONTH ___________________

<table>
<tr><td>MONDAY</td><td>SATURDAY</td></tr>
<tr><td>TUESDAY</td><td>SUNDAY</td></tr>
<tr><td>WEDNESDAY</td><td>SHOPPING LIST</td></tr>
<tr><td>THURSDAY</td><td></td></tr>
<tr><td>FRIDAY</td><td>NOTES:</td></tr>
</table>

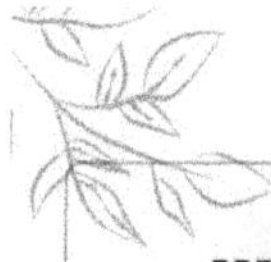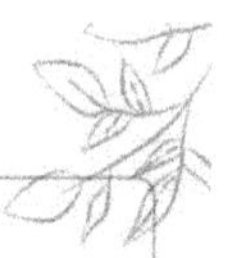

WEEKLY MEAL PLANNER JOURNAL

WEEK _______________   MONTH _______________

MONDAY

SATURDAY

TUESDAY

SUNDAY

WEDNESDAY

SHOPPING LIST

- ○ _______________
- ○ _______________
- ○ _______________
- ○ _______________
- ○ _______________
- ○ _______________
- ○ _______________
- ○ _______________

THURSDAY

FRIDAY

NOTES:

- ○ _______________
- ○ _______________
- ○ _______________
- ○ _______________

WEEKLY MEAL PLANNER JOURNAL

WEEK ___________________   MONTH ___________________

MONDAY

TUESDAY

WEDNESDAY

THURSDAY

FRIDAY

SATURDAY

SUNDAY

SHOPPING LIST

- ○ _______________________
- ○ _______________________
- ○ _______________________
- ○ _______________________
- ○ _______________________
- ○ _______________________
- ○ _______________________
- ○ _______________________

NOTES:

- ○ _______________________
- ○ _______________________
- ○ _______________________
- ○ _______________________

WEEKLY MEAL PLANNER JOURNAL

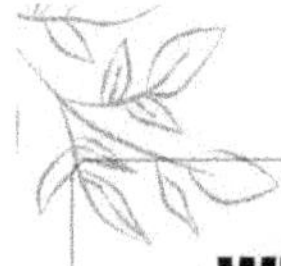
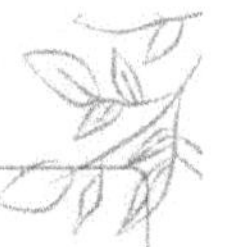

WEEK _______________________   MONTH _______________________

MONDAY

SATURDAY

TUESDAY

SUNDAY

WEDNESDAY

SHOPPING LIST

○ _______________________
○ _______________________
○ _______________________
○ _______________________
○ _______________________
○ _______________________
○ _______________________
○ _______________________

THURSDAY

FRIDAY

NOTES:

○ _______________________
○ _______________________
○ _______________________
○ _______________________

WEEKLY MEAL PLANNER JOURNAL

WEEK ___________________   MONTH ___________________

MONDAY

SATURDAY

TUESDAY

SUNDAY

WEDNESDAY

SHOPPING LIST

THURSDAY

FRIDAY

NOTES:

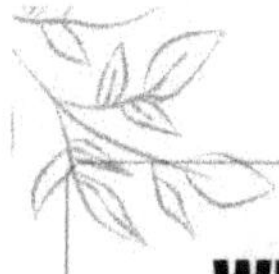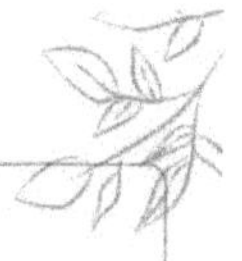

WEEKLY MEAL PLANNER JOURNAL

WEEK _______________________   MONTH _______________________

MONDAY

TUESDAY

WEDNESDAY

THURSDAY

FRIDAY

SATURDAY

SUNDAY

SHOPPING LIST

○ _______________________
○ _______________________
○ _______________________
○ _______________________
○ _______________________
○ _______________________
○ _______________________
○ _______________________

NOTES:

○ _______________________
○ _______________________
○ _______________________
○ _______________________

WEEKLY MEAL PLANNER JOURNAL

WEEK ________________________   MONTH ________________________

MONDAY

SATURDAY

TUESDAY

SUNDAY

WEDNESDAY

SHOPPING LIST

THURSDAY

FRIDAY

NOTES:

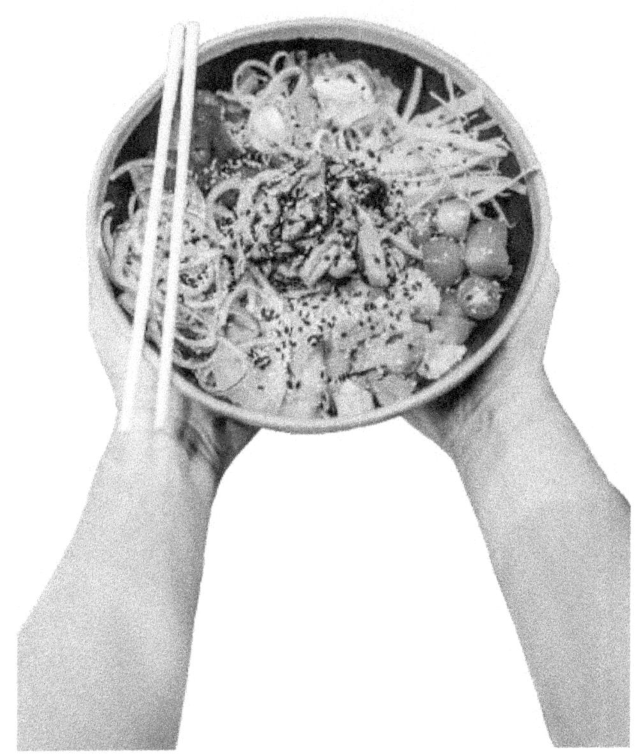

THANK YOU FOR READING!!!